3 – You Have Already Examined Your Other Options

As nice as it is to improve your appearance by undergoing a cosmetic surgery facelift, it is important to know that you do have other options. For example, scars or marks that resemble stretch marks can also be removed with laser surgery, as opposed to actually going under the knife. There are also a large number of over-the-counter products that are designed to help reduce wrinkles and slow down the signs of aging. Although surgery does produce quicker results, especially when compared to over-the-counter products, cosmetic surgery does cost more money.

4 – You Have Had Bad Reactions to Over-the-Counter Products

As it was previously stated, there are alternatives to cosmetic surgery facelifts. One of those alternatives is over-the-counter skincare products.

There are products that are designed for scars, acne, and wrinkles. Another sign that a surgical facelift may be in your best interest if you have tried a few of these over-the-counter products without success. In fact, have you had bad reactions to these products? Some consumers end up with even more skin problems, namely a bad case of skin irritation.

5 – You Want Results and You Want Them Now

Of course, when you undergo a surgical facelift, it is important to remember that you do need time to recover. Both your body and your skin will need to rest. When that rest and recovery time has ended, you should be able to see immediate results. Laser surgery often takes multiple sessions and over-the-counter skincare products need to be used for months before results are seen. So, if you want to improve the appearance of your face and see results right now, a surgical cosmetic facelift should be examined.

5 Signs You May Need a Cosmetic Surgery Facelift

Are you unhappy with the appearance of your face? Do you have scars, problems with acne, or is your face starting to show the early signs of aging? If so, you may be curious as to what all of your options are. Despite the fact that you do have a number of different treatment options, many men and women in your shoes opt for cosmetic surgery.

So, should you get a cosmetic surgery facelift? Of course, there are a number of factors that you will want to take into consideration when determining so. There are, however, signs that you will want to look for. If these signs, five of which are outlined below, apply to you, a cosmetic surgery facelift may be in your best interest.

1 – You Are Getting Older

It is no secret that our skin changes as we age. Unfortunately, these changes aren't always pleasant and attractive. Throughout the course of your life you may have developed small scars on your face. These can be taken care of with cosmetic surgery. Although there are a number of reasons why you could undergo a cosmetic surgery facelift, wrinkle treatment is the most common. It is important to remember that just because you are getting older in age; it doesn't mean that you have to look like it!

2 – You Are Embarrassed

Are you embarrassed by the way that you look? Although every single individual is beautiful in their own way, that may not help to change the way that you feel. Those who undergo cosmetic surgery facelifts often have the sole goal of improving their appearance. Whether you are depressed with the signs of aging, if your face is saggy-like after a large weight loss, or if you just want a change, a cosmetic surgery facelift may be an option for you to seriously consider.

The five above mentioned signs are just a few of the many signs that a cosmetic surgery facelift may be in your best interest. As a reminder, there are dangers that are associated with surgical facelifts, including pain and discomfort. Even with the possibility of painful side effects, many men and women, just like you, find that the pros outweigh the cons.

Common Cosmetic Surgery Alternatives

Are you interested in fixing an imperfection of yours? If you are, you may opt for cosmetic surgery. Cosmetic surgery is increasing in popularity, as many men and women are finding it an easy to improve the imperfections on their bodies.

As great as cosmetic surgery is, it is also important to look at it realistically. Unless your surgery is considered a reconstructive surgery or unless your health is at risk, like with gastric bypass surgery, there is a good chance that your health insurance will not cover your procedure. This means that you may be responsible for the full cost, which could be thousands of dollars!

It is also important to note that cosmetic surgery is a big deal. Whether you are simply just looking to reduce the appearance of your stretch marks or if you are looking to have a full body lift, cosmetic surgery is still a big deal. Although most surgeries are performed successfully, there are risks and dangers associated with seeking surgical treatment. For that reason, not everyone decides to move forward.

If you are unable to afford the cost of cosmetic surgery or if you don't feel like you can handle the whole process, you may be curious as to what your options are. If so, please continue reading on.

As it was previously stated, some individuals undergo cosmetic surgery to reduce the appearance of stretch marks. Similar steps are taken for those who are looking to reduce the appearance of scars, a tattoo, or a birthmark. Most often, you will not actually "go under the knife," but receive a laser surgery treatment instead. This is important to know if your main reason for avoiding surgery is fear.

As for your alternatives, when looking to improve the appearance of your skin, there are a number of over-the-counter skincare products that you can use. Although these skincare products will not remove a tattoo and although they cannot reduce the appearance of a birthmark, you can seek treatment for stretch marks, small scars, and wrinkles. You can visit your local drug store to examine a few of these products. Shopping and reading reviews online is nice as well. Typically, those with Vitamin E and Vitamin C are recommended for an improvement in appearance.

In keeping the appearance of the skin, if you are looking to remove unwanted hair, you do have a number of different options. In terms of unwanted hair removal, laser surgery is often performed. There are also a number of skincare products that can be purchased. Waxing and shaving are also two other options. If cost is not a concern of yours, electrolysis can be examined.

If you are looking to lose weight, you may opt for liposuction. Liposuction is ideal for those who are slightly overweight, but not obese. Those who suffer from obesity are encouraged to seek information on gastric bypass surgery. Although both types of surgery, gastric bypass and liposuction are advised, they can be somewhat painful and costly. The good news is that there are always ways that you can lose weight naturally. Although it may take some time getting use to, you can lose weight by creating and following a healthy meal plan and an exercise plan.

As you can see, you have several different options, as opposed to cosmetic surgery, when looking to lose weight, remove excess fat from your body, get rid of unwanted hair, as well as treat other skin imperfections. Speaking to your primary care physician is advised before deciding on a particular course of action.

Common Cosmetic Surgery Procedures

Have you recently decided that you would like to improve your physical appearance, namely by way of cosmetic surgery? If so, have you already decided on a course of treatment? Although a cosmetic surgeon can help you make your decision, there are a number of benefits to having a good idea of what you want before you attend a consultation appointment.

So, what type of cosmetic surgery should you undergo? If you still aren't sure yet, you may want to first take the time to familiarize yourself with some common procedures. To help get you started, a few of your surgical options are highlighted below and briefly summarized.

Mammoplasty is a term that is used to commonly describe cosmetic surgical procedures that are performed on the breasts. As for what these procedures are, there are three main ones. A breast lift involves the reshaping of the breasts. It is often performed to reduce the saggy skin that results from excess weight loss and aging. Breast augmentation, which is also commonly referred to as a breast enlargement, involves the use of implants, most often silicone, to increase breast size. On the other hand, breast reduction involves the reduction of tissue and skin to reduce the size of the breasts.

A facelift is another common cosmetic surgery procedure that is performed. Typically, those who are looking to reduce or completely eliminate their wrinkles and slow the signs of aging opt for facelifts. Cosmetic facelift surgeries are also commonly known as rhinoplasty.

Liposuction is another common cosmetic surgery procedure that is performed on men and women. Liposuction involves the removal of excess body fat from problem areas. These problem areas are typically the abdominal area, the thighs, and the underarms. Liposuction should not be confused with gastric bypass surgery and other similar procedures. These types of surgeries are often considered part of a weight loss plan, whereas liposuction isn't typically. With liposuction, a small amount of fat, usually between five to ten pounds, is removed.

When we often think of cosmetic surgery, the phrase "going under the knife," is often the first thing that comes to mind. While most cosmetic surgeries are considered invasive, not all require the breaking of the skin. This is thanks to laser surgery. Laser skin resurfacing is another common cosmetic procedure that is performed by qualified surgeons. Laser skin resurfacing is often use to smooth out imperfections, including small scars, stretch marks, wrinkles, and well as to remove tattoos or birthmarks. Laser surgery can also be used to remove unwanted hair, as well as to reduce the need for glasses and contacts.

In keeping with cosmetic procedures that don't involve actual cutting, there is that of chemical peels. Although chemical peels are offered by a number of establishments, including day spas, you may find the most comfort undergoing them at a qualified cosmetic surgery center. Chemical peels, as with laser skin resurfacing, can reduce the appearance of scars, wrinkles, stretch marks, and acne.

In addition to the above mentioned cosmetic surgery procedures, which focus on the body and skin in general, cosmetic dentistry should also be examined. After all, what good would a "new body," do if your teeth aren't up to standard? Cosmetic density is a field that is increasing in popularity, as more individuals start to take note of the health and appearance of their teeth. Common surgical procedures involved in cosmetic dentistry include the insertion of a dental implant and a gum lift.

As you can see, you have several different options when looking to improve your physical appearance by way of cosmetic surgery. What is even more amazing is that these are just a few of your options. Other areas that people, just like you, target include the buttocks, the chin, the checks, the eyelids, and the nose. As a reminder, a qualified cosmetic surgeon should be able to help you decide on the best course of action, so schedule a consultation appointment today.

Do you feel that your teeth are having a negative impact on your otherwise glowing smile? If you do, you may be interested in seeking treatment from a cosmetic dentist. Although there are a number of cosmetic dentistry procedures that you can undergo, a number of these procedures fall under the category of cosmetic surgery.

Although cosmetic dental surgery is generally considered safe, there are a still a number of risks. In fact, there are always dangers and risks when the skin or gums are broken. There is, however, something that you can do to protect yourself. By carefully choosing your cosmetic dentist, you are likely to see the best results, as well as a decrease in complication risks.

In keeping with choosing the right cosmetic dentist, you may have the option of staying with your primary care dentist. There are many dentists who also perform cosmetic procedures, including veneers, teeth whitening, dental implants, and gum lifts. With that said, be sure to inquire about the success rate and frequency of those procedures. You may feel more comfortable visiting a dentist who performs cosmetic surgery procedures on a daily basis, as opposed to a few times a month.

As for how you can go about finding a cosmetic dentist, you may want ask your primary care dentist for recommendations. Let them know that you will return to their offices for your annual checkups, but that you feel more comfortable seeing a specialist. They should understand your decision and even give you recommendations. In addition to asking your primary care dentist, ask any friends, coworkers, or family members if they know of any quality cosmetic dentists in the area.

Although the above-mentioned steps can help you find cosmetic dentists in your area, you need to choose a dentist. Simply just picking one out of the phone book can increase your chances of poor results and complications. Instead, you will want to do the proper amount of research online. This is easy if your local cosmetic dentists have online websites. On those websites, you will likely find information on cosmetic procedures performed, a brief summary of the process, average rates, as well as before and after pictures. Also, be sure to examine qualifications and the number of years in dentistry.

Cost should also be examined. Cosmetic surgery isn't always covered by dental insurance, but you may be surprised to know that some procedures are. Many insurance companies find veneers an affordable way to reduce the long-term costs of dental care. Dental implants are also a nice alternative to dentures. Do not make the assumption that your insurance does not cover cosmetic procedures until you know for sure. On the back of your dental insurance card, you should see a customer service phone number that you can call to make the inquiry.

Once you have decided that you would like to improve your smile with the use of a cosmetic dental procedure, you will want to schedule a consultation appointment. Most dentists do require them; however, still ask for a consultation appointment even if they are only optional. At a consultation appointment, you and your cosmetic dentist can decide on a course of treatment, highlight the procedures you will undergo in detail, summarize the recovery process, as well as show you sample before and after pictures.

Cosmetic Surgery Abroad: Is It Really Cheaper?

Are you looking to undergo cosmetic surgery? Regardless of what type of procedure you are looking to have, whether it be liposuction or a facelift, you may be concerned with cost. In fact, cost is a concern of many hopeful cosmetic surgery patients.

Affordable prices and cosmetic surgery aren't always two things that are associated with each other. That is why those who are on a budget often examine cosmetic surgery abroad. You may be doing the same thing, but is it really cheaper? In all honesty, yes and no.

Although a mixed answer isn't likely what you wanted to hear, it is the truth. There are a number of qualified cosmetic surgeons overseas who are known for producing quality, amazing, and flawless results. The only difference, in some cases, is that the surgical procedures do not cost the same. This is due to the fact the cost of living has an impact on the sale of services and goods. Since the cost of living in the United States is quite high, many individuals, like you like, look abroad.

Although you may be able to find cheap cosmetic surgery procedures, like liposuction, facelifts, and excess skin removal, available abroad, there are some important points that you will first want to take into consideration. These points, a few of which are outlined below, should be examined before you start making your travel arrangements and before you officially book your appointment.

The overall cost of undergoing cosmetic surgery abroad should be examined. You need to examine more than just the cost of surgery. What about the cost and the time that it will take to get a passport? The cost of airline reservations should also be examined. How do you intend to travel once you arrive at your destination? Examine the cost of public transportation or the cost of renting a car.

It is also extremely important that you examine the length of your stay. Some cosmetic procedures, including full body lifts, aren't just get up and run procedures. You may need to return to have a post-surgery checkup, return for additional work, or you may have to return if complications arise. This can impact your cost of travel, as well as the length of your trip. How long will you need to stay at a hotel? How much work will you end up missing?

Perhaps, the greatest point that needs to be taken into consideration, when examining cosmetic surgery abroad, is safety. As it was previously stated, there are some cosmetic surgeons abroad who do produce flawless results, but the others can do more damage to your body. Not all countries have the same medical standards, rules, and restrictions that the United States does. This means that there is an increased chance of complications, including a staph infection from unclean instruments.

If you do opt for cosmetic surgery abroad, it is important that you do the proper amount of research first. You can use the internet. Once you have the name of the surgeon who would perform your surgery, perform a standard internet search with the name. Are there any complaints or warnings posted online? If so, it may be best to examine other abroad surgeons or even stay closer to home. In fact, you may simply just want to target the largest city that is closest to your home. This should give you more options, qualifications, and prices to choose from.

Cosmetic Surgery and Teens: Is It a Good Idea?

Are you the parent of a teenager who has recently decided that they would like to undergo cosmetic surgery? If so, you may be feeling a wide array of emotions right now. Although most parents in your shoes wouldn't even entertain the thought, you may be interested in doing so. You may be curious as to whether or not cosmetic surgery and teens go together.

As for whether or not cosmetic surgery is advised for teenagers, it will all depend. All teenagers are not the same. Cosmetic surgery procedures are performed for a wide range of reasons. To help you determine if your teenager is ready for cosmetic surgery, there are a number of factors that you will first want to take into consideration.

For starters, it is important to examine your child's health. Is your child's health at risk if they do not undergo cosmetic surgery? For example, is your child seriously obese? If so, gastric bypass surgery or other weight loss surgeries may be needed. Of course, as a parent, you owe it to your child to help them explore other options. You and your teenager may first want to try more natural ways of losing weight, such as eating healthy and exercising regularly.

Since most cosmetic surgery procedures are performed with the sole purpose of improving appearance, you may not understand why your teenager needs treatment. Be sure to talk to your child about their reasoning. Are they being harassed at school? Does your child have a skin growth or unwanted body hair that is resulting in them getting teased at school? If so, you may want to inquire about cosmetic surgery. It is important to know the impact that constant harassment and heckling can have on a teenager's self-confidence and self-esteem.

Before getting your child's heart set on cosmetic surgery, if you do voice your approval, you will first want to make sure that your child is even a good candidate. Do you know that some cosmetic surgeons will not perform surgical procedures on those under the age of 18? Others do have restrictions, but may be a little bit more lax with them. For example, ideal candidates for liposuction are over the age of 18. This is often due in part to the maturity levels.

Speaking of maturity, is your child mature enough to make a well-informed decision about cosmetic surgery? Most teenagers aren't. Many just know that they want to look beautiful, no matter what the costs. Can your child handle those costs though? If your child is thinking about cosmetic surgery just to improve their beauty, it may be a wise idea to let them make their own decision when they turn 18.

Another reason why not all teenagers are ideal candidates for cosmetic surgery is because of the recovery process. If breast reduction is performed, your child will need to get the proper amount of rest. They may also face certain restrictions, such as no heavy lifting or no wearing a bra for a week. Will your teenager be able to follow their post surgery directions right down to the letter? If not, they may end up hurting their health and the results of their surgery.

As a reminder, many cosmetic surgeons in the United States have restrictions and rules set for cosmetic surgery and minors. If you do opt for cosmetic surgery for your teen, schedule a consultation appointment with them to see if they are an ideal candidate.

Cosmetic Surgery and Weight Loss

Are you looking to lose weight? If you are, you may also be looking for a little bit of help. Cosmetic surgery is often performed to improve one's physical appearance, but there are certain situations in which it could actually be a lifesaver.

These situations often involve those who are overweight.

One of the most sought after cosmetic procedures performed is that of liposuction. Liposuction is designed to remove excess fat from the body. Often times, specific "problem," areas are targeted. Common areas on both men and women include the underarms, the thighs, and the abdominal area.

If you are interested in undergoing liposuction, it is important to know that you may not necessarily get to. Quality cosmetic surgeons, namely the ones you will want operating on you, have strict standards and qualifications for candidates. These typically include those of the age of eighteen, those in good health, and those who have the desire to lose weight. Good health and the desire to stay on a healthy path is important so that complications do not arise.

Unfortunately, those who are obese aren't always good candidates for liposuction. This is because only a small about of fat can be removed at once, as there are dangers to removing too much. Also, those who are obese are likely to have diabetes, high blood pressure, and heart problems. These all increase the risk of complications. If you are obese, there is good new though. You may be a candidate for gastric bypass surgery or another similar procedure, like the Lapband. Your primary care physician may be able to help you determine which surgery you are the best candidate for.

In addition to assisting with weight loss, cosmetic surgery can also be used to help those who have lost a significant amount of weight. If you had a large weight loss, like 100 pounds or more, you may have a lot of excess skin just, literally, hanging around. This may make you feel unattractive and scared to show off your great new body. It is ironic when this happens though, as one of your weight loss goals was to look good. Cosmetic surgery, as previously stated, can provide you with assistance. You can receive a full body lift, unless you have specific areas you would like targeted. Although there are a number of side effects, including pain and discomfort, you will likely be pleased with the results.

As a reminder, not everyone is the perfect candidate for cosmetic surgery. The first thing that you will want to do is find and choose a cosmetic surgeon or surgery center in your area. You can then schedule a consultation appointment for yourself. At this appointment, you will have the procedure explained to you and your surgeon will help you decide if cosmetic surgery is the best option for you.

Before proceeding too far, it is also important to examine the cost. If you are without health insurance, you will have to pay for the full costs of your surgery. Even if you are insured, you may still be responsible for the cost. Most cosmetic procedures, like liposuction and the removal of excess skin, are not covered. With that said, gastric bypass surgery and other similar procedures are about more than just improving physical appearance, as they can often be a lifesaver.

Cosmetic Surgery Before and After Pictures: Why You Should Examine Them

Are you thinking about undergoing cosmetic surgery? Cosmetic surgery is a phrase that covers a wide range of surgical procedures. Whether you are looking to have unwanted body hair removed or get a full body lift, you may be unsure about your decision. You may have a ton of questions. One easy way that you can get answers to many of those questions is by examining cosmetic surgery before and after pictures.

As nice as it is to hear that you should examine cosmetic surgery before and after pictures, you may be curious as to why you should and how you can do so. If that is what you are wondering, please continue reading on.

One of the many reasons why you should examine cosmetic surgery before and after pictures is because they can give you a good idea as to what you can expect. Although you know that a facelift can be used to reduce or eliminate wrinkles, as well as slow the signs of aging, you may not know what the end result will actually look like. This, however, is something that you need to know.

In addition to giving you an idea as to what you can expect, when undergoing cosmetic surgery, examining before and after pictures can help to make sure that you are being realistic. As previously stated, a surgical facelift can reduce wrinkles and the signs of aging, but that doesn't necessarily mean that your face will look the same as it did when you were twenty years old. Unfortunately, those with unrealistic expectations often find themselves disappointed and that is not how you should be feeling after cosmetic surgery.

Cosmetic surgery before and after pictures can also help provide you with reassurance that you did choose the best surgeon in your area. For that to happen, you need to make sure that you are shown before and after pictures from procedures that your surgeon performed. Make sure that you ask, as some cosmetic surgery centers have been known to use standard, generic photographs.

As for how you can find cosmetic surgery before and after pictures to examine, you do have a number of different options. Inquire at your local cosmetic surgery center or at the office of a private practice. They should have before and after pictures for you to examine. You may have to examine them there. Remember to make sure that the pictures are of those where the surgery was performed on site. Also, make sure the before and after pictures are of the procedure you wish to undergo, like liposuction or a surgical facelift.

You can also use the internet to find cosmetic surgery before and after pictures to examine. For starters, you may want to visit the online websites of your local cosmetic surgeons or surgical centers. This will give you the time to examine the same pictures at your own pace and in the comfort of your own home. Additional pictures can be found with a standard internet search. When doing so, use a phrase like "liposuction before and after pictures." This approach is easy, but remember that surgeons do produce different results.

As a recap, examining before and after pictures of cosmetic surgeries, namely the procedure you plan to undergo, can give you an idea of what you can expect in terms of results. Since these pictures are easy to find, there is no reason why you should go in for surgery without having realistic expectations.

Cosmetic Surgery: How to Protect Yourself

Are you interested in undergoing cosmetic surgery? If you are, you may already know what specific procedure you would like to undergo. However, you may not yet have had the chance to choose a cosmetic surgeon or a cosmetic surgery center. If that is the case, you will want to proceed with caution, as you will want to protect yourself.

For starters, it is important to know that cosmetic surgery does have risks and dangers. That is why you will want to protect yourself. While you may automatically think of your health, there are other aspects of yourself that you will want to protect as well.

As previously stated, you will want to protect your health when undergoing cosmetic surgery. Although not always common, complications during surgery may arise. Unfortunately, one of those complications may be death. Also, staph infections of the skin can be common after surgery. That is why you will want to make sure that you choose a well-known cosmetic surgeon or center with a good reputation. This will help to make sure that your health is protected, as the practice and their surgical instruments are clean.

In keeping with protecting your health, it is also important to examine after surgery care. Unfortunately, this is something that many patients do not take into consideration until it is too late. Do not make this mistake. Will you be able to follow all after surgery directions to given to you? If not, you, yourself, may end up causing a skin infection or other similar complications. That is why you must be sure that you can handle the recovery process, no matter how short or long it will be, before you go in for the procedure.

In addition to protecting your health, you also need to protect your appearance. Despite the fact that cosmetic surgery turns out good the majority of the time, there are cases of serious errors being made. These errors often result in unattractiveness that can be hard and costly to fix. This, however, can be prevented. When looking to undergo cosmetic surgery, you can protect yourself by carefully choosing your cosmetic surgeon or cosmetic surgery center.

As for how you should choose a cosmetic surgeon or cosmetic surgical center, you can do the research locally and online. You can perform a standard internet search with the name of the doctor you would like more information on. What do you see online? Ask those in the waiting room or others that you know if they have any feedback. If you are visiting a surgical center, where multiple doctors are, be sure to get the name of the surgeon who will be performing your procedure. Make sure that they have a good reputation, a strong background in the surgical field, and that they produce good results.

While it is most important to protect your health and appearance, when looking to undergo cosmetic surgery, you also need to protect your wallet. Cosmetic surgery, as you likely already know, can be very costly. Unless you are undergoing a procedure, like breast reduction or gastric bypass surgery, there is a good chance that your health insurance will not cover the cost. This means that you will need to do so yourself.

In keeping with protecting your wallet, you will not want to overpay for your cosmetic surgery procedure. For that reason, you are urged to compare prices. In addition to comparing prices, remember to compare success rates and reputation. As important as it is to protect your wallet, your health, appearance, and safety should not be comprised just so that you can get a good deal.

As you can see, there are a number of risks that are associated with cosmetic surgery, but remember that there are also steps that you can take to protect yourself. Never go in for surgery without first knowing as much as you can about the procedure, the recovery process, the full costs, and the surgeon doing the job.

Cosmetic Surgery in Larger Cities: Why It May Be Best

Have you recently made the decision to undergo cosmetic surgery? If you have, that decision, alone, is a large one, but you have one more important decision to make. That decision is which cosmetic surgeon or surgery center you want to visit. You may have heard that you should target those located in big cities, but is that really true? Yes and no.

As previously stated, there is some truth the claim that you can find the best luck with searching for a cosmetic surgery center or a surgeon with a private practice in larger cities. With that said, it honestly all depends. Who do you have available locally? Even if you live in a small town or city, did you know that the one cosmetic surgeon that you do have may have outstanding credentials, a large amount of experience, as well as a high success rate of producing beautiful, satisfied patients? That is why you should first examine your options locally.

As for why it is a good idea for you to examine cosmetic surgeons in a nearby, larger city, it will give you access to more doctors with private practices. These are professionals who work by themselves, but with a small team of qualified nurses. Logical thinking proves that the larger the area you are in the more you will find, and the same applies to cosmetic surgeons.

In addition to finding more cosmetic surgeons with private practices, you also stand a chance of finding more cosmetic surgery centers to choose from. This automatically gives you access to more doctors. On average, a cosmetic surgery center has around two or three surgeons on staff. If you do choose this option, be sure that you get the name of the professional who will be performing your procedure ahead of time. This will give you the appropriate amount of time to review their qualifications, their reputation, as well as their success rate.

By examining cosmetic surgeons and cosmetic surgery centers in a larger city, you open yourself up to a larger range of procedures. When most of us hear the phrase "cosmetic surgery," being cut open is often the first thought that comes to mind. Yes, liposuction and body lifts do involve the use of a scalpel; however, there are other procedures that don't. These procedures include chemical peels and laser surgery. Unfortunately, not all private practices and cosmetic surgery centers offer them, but your chances do increase in a larger city.

By examining cosmetic surgery centers and private practice surgeons in a larger city, you are likely to find the best rates. Since you do have a number of different options, be sure to compare rates. This is great and it may even be necessary if you don't have any health insurance or if your health insurance does not cover cosmetic surgery. Speaking of which, be sure to check. There are a small number of cosmetic surgeries that some health insurance providers do cover, like breast reduction. In keeping with prices, don't make the mistake of automatically going with the cheapest that you can find. Quality and fees should be examined together.

So, what is the best option for you? It all depends. First, take a close look at where you live. How many surgery centers or private practice cosmetic surgeons do you have within a half an hours drive?

If only one or two, you should examine the closest big city. Remember that you should do more than just find a cosmetic surgeon; you should also choose one. For this to happen though, you must first have a choice.

As for how you can make your choice, there are a number of factors that you will want to take into consideration. Despite the fact that results will vary, examining before and after pictures can give you a good idea of what you can expect. Make sure the pictures aren't generic, but of procedures that your surgeon has actually performed. Examine his or her success rate, as well as the rate of complications.

Cosmetic Surgery Patient Stories: Why You Should First Read Them

Are you in the process of considering cosmetic surgery? If you are, you may be looking for more information. After all, the decision to undergo cosmetic surgery is a big decision; it is not one that should be made on a whim. If you are interested in undergoing cosmetic surgery to correct an imperfection, such as excess skin, excess fat, stretch marks, or winkles, but are not one hundred percent sure about your decision, you may be unsure as to how you should proceed. For starters, you may want to examine cosmetic surgery patient stories.

Cosmetic surgery patient stores, as you likely already know, are stories that are told by those who have undergone cosmetic surgery. They are firsthand accounts, which are often posted online. If you haven't already taken the time to read a few of these firsthand accounts you will want to do so. Most importantly, you will want to do so before you make your final decision about your surgery.

As for what reading cosmetic surgery patient stories can do for you, it can help you understand the reasoning behind these popular surgeries. Although you may want to slow the signs of aging and eliminate your wrinkles, you may be wondering if cosmetic surgery is really your best option. By examining cosmetic surgery patient stories, you can see that people undergo cosmetic surgery for a number of different reasons. These are people just like you and many have the same reasons for choosing surgery. This may help to provide you with reassurance that you are making the right decision.

Cosmetic surgery patient stories can help you know what to expect. For the best results, you will want to read the firsthand accounts of those who underwent the procedure that you are interested in, like a surgical facelift. Many patients will tell you how the procedure worked, often in a step-by-step format. They may also outline what they were feeling at the time, whether it be fear or excitement, as well as share ways on how to cope with those emotions.

The recovery process is an important component of undergoing a successful cosmetic surgery procedure. Unfortunately, many do not know just how important the recovery process is. Should you choose to go forward with the procedure, you will likely receive a set of instructions. These instructions may include having your area covered with bandages, applying antibiotic ointment, and so forth. In addition to outlining what the recovery process entails, the side effects, such as slight pain and discomfort, may also be touched on.

Perhaps, the greatest reason why you should find and read cosmetic surgery patient stories is because you can learn how cosmetic surgery changed the lives of others just like you. Once again, this can help you determine if cosmetic surgery is really in your best interest. Although you will find varied accounts, those who undergo surgery often report an improvement in health, an improvement in physical appearance, and an improvement in self-esteem and self-confidence. These are the same improvements that you too can experience.

As for how you can find cosmetic surgery patient stories, there are a number of different approaches that you can take. They are easier to find online. You can perform a standard internet search. Many cosmetic surgery centers also post stories and testimonials on their websites. Your local surgical centers may also have similar information available for your viewing in print.

In addition to reading firsthand accounts from other surgery patients, who are essentially strangers, you may want to ask those that you know. If any of your friends, relatives, coworkers, or neighbors have undergone a cosmetic procedure, inquire about their experience. Since cosmetic procedures, like breast reductions and facelifts, do vary, you may want to try to speak with those who have undergone the same surgical procedure. This approach is nice as you can also ask any additional questions that you may have.

Cosmetic Surgery Recovery: The Importance of Following All Directions

Did you just recently schedule an appointment to undergo cosmetic surgery? Regardless of what type of procedure you are having, recovery time is important. In fact, your cosmetic surgeon should provide you with a set of post-surgery directions for you to follow. Do you know just how important it is that you follow those directions?

Simply just knowing that it is important to follow all post-surgery directions isn't enough for many individuals. Many are often left wondering what the worst is that could happen. In all honesty, if you really did know there is a good chance that you won't miss a step, no matter how large or small, in your recovery process.

As for the dangers or risks that are associated with not following all post-surgery directions that are given to you, the greatest is the risk of complications. If you undergo liposuction or have excess skin removed from your body, cutting will be involved. Of course, you will be closed back up, but did you know that wounds are subject to infection? Many are. That is why you should proceed with caution. Skin infections that result from improper care aren't only painful, but they can cause serious health complications, including the early onset of death.

Another reason why it is important for you to follow the directions given to you by your cosmetic surgeon for the recovery process is because of results. There are some cosmetic procedures, like liposuction and gastric bypass surgery, where certain steps must be taken by you. For liposuction, excess fat, around five to ten pounds, will be removed from your problem spots. To keep your lean look, you must be able to eat healthy and start a regular exercise plan. If you do not abide by your doctor's instructions to do so, you may gain the weight and excess fat back in as little as a few months. This, essentially, means that you wasted your money on surgery in the first place.

As previously stated, your cosmetic surgeon should provide you with a detailed list of directions to follow after your surgery. In fact, this information should be discussed ahead of time, during your consultation appointment. If you have yet to have your consultation appointment, you may be curious as to what the recovery process will be like for you. Typically, it will depend on what specific procedure you will undergo; however, there are some common steps that can and should be taken.

Over-the-counter pain medicines can be used for the slight pain and discomfort you are likely to experience from cosmetic surgery. Be sure to inquire as to which medications are the best. An ice pack will likely need to be applied to help reduce the swelling. You may also be required to change your bandages daily or keep them clean and dry until your next visit. You will also likely face restrictions. For body work, like liposuction, breast enlargements and reductions, you may be required to avoid heavy lifting and exercising for at least two to three weeks.

As you can see, it is important that you follow any after surgery instructions provided to you by your cosmetic surgeon. If you have any questions or concerns about the recovery process, please ask and before your procedure begins. In fact, make sure that you have any lingering questions answered at your consultation appointment.

Cosmetic Surgery versus Reconstructive Surgery

Are you interested in improving your physical appearance by way of surgery? If you are, you may turn to the internet to learn more. When examining surgical procedures online, you will find information on cosmetic surgeries and reconstructive surgeries. If you are like many others, you may be wondering if there is a difference between the two.

Although they are both similar in nature, there is a difference between cosmetic surgery and reconstructive surgery. Determining which type of surgery you need to undergo is important, as it may have an impact on the amount that you have to pay.

As for reconstructive surgery, it is surgery that is performed to repair or correct the body. Many parents seek surgery for their children who are born with birth defects. A common example of this is the correction of oversized ears. Diseases and other illnesses that cause damage to the body can also be repaired with reconstructive surgery. For example, women with breast cancer may have to undergo a mastectomy. To correct the unevenness that is left, patients often have their breasts restored to as close as normal with surgery.

In addition to correcting birth defects and other abnormalities, reconstructive surgery is also used to treat and help accident victims recover. Burn victims undergo reconstructive surgery to repair their scar tissue. Car accident victims and victims of other similar accidents may need to undergo reconstructive surgery to repair a crushed bone or to have a limb reattached.

Unlike reconstructive surgery, cosmetic surgery does not correct abnormities. Instead, the main goal of cosmetic surgery is to improve one's appearance. With cosmetic surgery, patients can and likely would lead a normal life even without treatment.

As with reconstructive surgery, there are a number of procedures that are considered cosmetic. These procedures include abdominoplasty (tummy tuck), mammoplasty (breast reduction, breast enlargement, breast lift), rhinoplasty (nose job), liposuction, and rhytidectomy (facelift). As previously stated, cosmetic surgery is optional. Many individuals choose to undergo cosmetic surgery to improve their physical appearance. These individuals are usually embarrassed about an imperfection that they have, such as unwanted body hair or excessive wrinkling of the face.

As for the cost of these surgeries, cosmetic surgery is rarely covered by a traditional health insurance plan. That doesn't mean you shouldn't make an inquiry however. As for reconstructive surgery, a good percentage of procedures are covered. This, as previously stated, is because those undergoing reconstructive surgery often aren't given an option. Cosmetic surgery, on the other hand, is an optional procedure that patients should cover the cost of if they want and choose to have it.

Now that you know that there is a significant difference between cosmetic surgery and reconstructive surgery, which type of surgery do you need to seek? In addition to having an impact on costs, it may also have an impact on your treatment options.

If your insurance is covering the cost of reconstructive surgery, you may be required to visit your local hospital, as opposed to a cosmetic surgery center. In fact, you should first have answers to this important question. If you are responsible for the full cost of your surgery, whether it be cosmetic or reconstructive, be sure to wisely make your choice. Choose those with affordable fees, but with outstanding qualifications and a significant amount of experience in the field.

How and Why You Should Use the Internet to Research Cosmetic Surgery

Are you thinking about undergoing cosmetic surgery? No matter what type of procedure you are looking to undergo and regardless of your reasons for doing so, it is important that you first do your research. The good news is that this research is easy to do online.

Before focusing on ways that you can use the internet to research cosmetic surgery, you may be curious as to why you should do so. For starters, you may have already decided that you want to undergo cosmetic surgery, but what are your reasons for doing so? Are they good? Do you have any other alternatives? Although cosmetic surgery will likely provide you with the results you were looking for, as the success rate is very high, do you know that there are still dangers and risks associated with it?

Now that you know just a few of the many reasons why you should take the time to research cosmetic surgery online, you may be curious as to how you can go about doing so. The good news is that you do have a number of different options.

First, you are urged to perform a standard internet search with the phrase "cosmetic surgery dangers." There are dangers and risks associated with surgery and they are important to know. Typically, you will find information on how cosmetic surgeons can make errors, how you may have a bad reaction to the anesthesia, or how you are at risk for developing an infection if you don't properly follow your recovery instructions.

If you are still interested in undergoing cosmetic surgery, even after knowing the dangers and risks associated with doing so, you will want to learn more about your procedure. Cosmetic surgery encompasses a number of different procedures. For that reason, you will want to perform a standard internet search with the specific procedure you are interested in having, like liposuction, a face life, or breast enlargement. The websites that you find will likely be medical in nature. They should give you valuable information, including information on what steps will be performed during the procedure, as well as what the recovery process will be like for you.

Learning as much as you can about the cosmetic surgery procedure you are about to undergo is extremely important. Why? Because it can help you determine if it is really something that you can handle. For example, if you are required to change your bandages or apply antibiotic ointment to your spot three times a day, will you be able to do so?

It is also a good idea to examine before and after pictures online. What you will want to do is perform a standard internet search with this or a similar phrase "liposuction before and after pictures." If possible, examine before and after pictures from the cosmetic surgery center or surgeon you are interested in seeking treatment from. This can also give you an idea as to what type of individual results you should expect from them.

Finally, it is a good idea to read cosmetic surgery patients stories online. These stores are often found on the online websites of cosmetic surgery centers, but they can also be found with a standard internet search. Reading patient stories gives you a unique, inside look at cosmetic surgery. Patients often share their reasons for undergoing cosmetic surgery, what the procedure was like, how the recovery process went, as well as whether or not they were satisfied with the results.

It is also important to note that you can use the internet to find and research a cosmetic surgery center or a cosmetic surgeon in your area. When doing so, you have two main options. You can perform a standard internet search similar to this one "New York cosmetic surgeons," or you can use an online business directory. As an important side not, do not just pick the first surgeon that you come across. Instead, research their fees, examine their success rate, and their background in the surgical field.

How Cosmetic Surgery Can Improve Your Life

Are you concerned or constantly distracted with an imperfection that your body may have? If you just lost a lot of weight, excess skin may be causing you to feel ashamed and embarrassed. Wrinkles, due the early signs of aging, and unwanted body hair are just a few of the many imperfections that individuals, just like you, want to treat. The good news is that you likely have a number of different options, including cosmetic surgery.

As nice as it is to hear that cosmetic surgery is an option that you can choose, you may be unsure if it is the right decision. With the costs and the risks, many individuals wonder if the impact that cosmetic surgery will have on their life is really worth it. For you to make a decision, you should first review a few of the many ways that cosmetic surgery can improve your life.

For starters, it is important to examine your self-confidence and self-esteem. If you have an imperfection on your body that is easily visible to others, like unwanted body hair that just won't stay away, your self-confidence may be poor. Other than that unwanted hair, you may feel beautiful and attractive. Once the problem is taken care of you, you are likely to notice an improvement in your self-worth, self-confidence, and self-esteem. For many individuals, this is more than worth the costs of cosmetic surgery.

Along with an improvement in self-confidence and an improvement in self-esteem comes the ability to socialize better. Those with noticeable body or skin imperfections, even small, often hide themselves from others out of fear of being embarrassed or poorly judged. The good news is that if you use cosmetic surgery to seek treatment, you don't have to hide or live in fear of embarrassment any longer. If you are currently single, you may enjoy spending more time with your friends or even approaching others for dates!

Even if you are not single, but married, there is still a lot that cosmetic surgery can do for you. There comes a point in just about every marriage where husbands and wives reach a comfort zone. One of the first things to go is appearance. Cosmetic surgery can help to make your spouse fall in love with you all over again, like it was when you first met. Also, the increase in self-worth and self-confidence, which was touched on above, may do wonders for your marriage, namely where sex and communication is involved.

Cosmetic surgery, depending on what type of procedure you are looking to undergo, may also give you an advantage in the working world. Do you have poor teeth? Could you use a visit to a cosmetic dentist? Veneers, teeth whitening, dental implants, and gum lifts are common cosmetic procedures that will give you a happy, healthy, and professional smile. While we should be judged on our qualifications in the workplace, you may be surprised to learn just how big of an impact appearance does have.

As you can see, there are a number of different ways that undergoing cosmetic surgery can help to improve your life. If you are ready to get started, contact one of your local cosmetic surgeons or surgery centers today to schedule a consultation appointment. During this appointment, your physician can work with you to determine if you are an ideal candidate for cosmetic surgery, as well discuss your procedural options.

How to Find a Cosmetic Surgery Center

Have you recently decided that you would like to undergo cosmetic surgery? Regardless of whether you are looking to undergo liposuction, get a facelift, or have your excess skin removed, you will want and need to find a quality cosmetic surgery center with a good reputation to do the job.

One of the best ways to find a quality cosmetic surgery center to seek treatment from is by speaking to your primary care physician. If you are unable to do so, consider calling or stopping by your local hospital. In the medical field, most doctors have an open network of communication. This means that your primary care physician or hospital workers should be able to give you the contact information of local cosmetic surgery centers or surgeons with their own private practices. This approach is nice, as you won't get sent to just anyone.

Another easy way that you can go about finding a local cosmetic surgery center is by using the internet. When doing so, you have a couple of different options. For starters, you will want to perform a standard internet search. Be sure to incorporate your location into your search, like by using the phrases "Atlanta cosmetic surgery," or "Atlanta cosmetic surgery centers." Your standard internet search should connect you with practices that have online websites. You can view these online websites to get more information, as well as contact information.

In keeping with using the internet, you can also use online business directories to find local cosmetic surgery centers or surgeons with their own private practices. Many search engines have business directory features that you are able to use. What you will want to do is search for the type of business that you are looking for, a cosmetic surgery center, and then your location. You should be provided with an address and telephone number for each of your results.

Speaking of phone numbers, you can also use your local phone book to find cosmetic surgeons with private practices or cosmetic surgery centers. In the back of your phone book should be a business directory section, which is also commonly referred to as the yellow pages. Under the heading of physicians, you should find information on cosmetic surgeons. If your phone book does not automatically categorize physicians based on their specialty, look for headings that contain the phrases "cosmetic," or "cosmetic surgery."

Another great approach that you can take is to ask those that you know for recommendations. Cosmetic surgery is increasing in popularity. For that reason, there is a good chance that you know someone who has gone under the knife, even for a simple procedure like the removal of a mole. Ask your friends, family members, neighbors, or coworkers if they know of any quality cosmetic surgeons or cosmetic surgery centers in your area. Asking for recommendations from those that you know is nice because it limits the amount of research that you have to do yourself.

As for why you should do research, it is important to remember that there are a number of dangers and risks that are associated with cosmetic surgery. For that reason, you need to make sure that you choose a well-qualified cosmetic surgeon. By taking the time to find the best surgeon or surgical center in your area, you are likely to reduce the chances of complications, as well as improve your chances of getting the results you were hoping for. The last thing that you will want to do is choose the first surgeon that you come across. When undergoing cosmetic, it is important to make sure that you take steps to protect your health, your appearance, and your wallet.

Now that you know just a few of the many ways that you can go about finding cosmetic surgeons in your area, you can get started. Remember to do the proper amount of research first. In fact, you may want to schedule a couple of consultation appointments with different surgeons before making your final decision.

How to Find a Cosmetic Surgery Dentist

Are you interested in improving your smile? Sometimes, a simple cavity filling isn't enough. If you need a considerable amount of work done on your teeth, you may want to schedule an appointment with a cosmetic dentist. Although your primary care dentist may be able to provide you with assistance, cosmetic dentistry is often considered a completely different medical field.

As more individuals become concerned with the appearance of their teeth, cosmetic dentistry is increasing in popularity. For that reason, you should have a number of local cosmetic dentists to choose from. Do you know how you can find them though?

One of the easiest ways to find a cosmetic dentist is to ask your primary care dentist. Even if your dentist can perform the procedure that you are looking for more information on, like dental implants, he or she will still likely understand and respect your decision to seek care from a specialist. Asking your primary dentist for information and feedback on area cosmetic dentists, especially those that specialize in surgical procedures, is nice, as you likely won't be sent to just anyone.

The internet is another easy way that you can go about finding local cosmetic dentists. To get you started, you may want to use online business directories, which are typically provided by search engines. You can search for a specific type of business, like a cosmetic dentist, and your location, like Atlanta. The information that you will be provided with may vary, but you should get the names, addresses, and telephone numbers of cosmetic dentists in or around your immediate area.

In keeping with using the internet to find a cosmetic dentist, namely one that specializes in surgical procedures, you can perform a standard internet search. When doing so, your search phrase should look like this "Atlanta cosmetic dentist." Your internet search will likely lead you to the online websites of area dentists. Not only should you use these websites to get contact information, but also examine them for sample rates, lists of procedures performed, as well as before and after pictures.

Your local phone book can also be used to find area cosmetic dentists. What you will want to do is turn to the back of your phone book. Here, you will find a business directory section, which is also commonly known as the yellow pages of the phone book. Under the heading of dentists, you should see information on your local options. Unless your local phone book categorizes dentists, like pediatric dentists and cosmetic dentists, look for listings with the word "cosmetic," in them.

Aside from asking your primary dentist for suggestions, your next best option is to speak with those that you know. Ask your friends, relatives, neighbors, or coworkers if they have ever been to a cosmetic dentist before. If they have, who did they visit? Were they satisfied with the results? Does he or she charge affordable rates? Getting recommendations from those that you know will lessen the amount of background and reputation checking and you will have to do yourself.

As an important reminder, you will want to do more than find a cosmetic dentist who specializes in surgical procedures. You will want to actually choose one. When making your choice, examine fees, qualifications, before and after pictures, and success rate versus complication rate.

How to Pay for Your Cosmetic Surgery

Have you recently decided that you would like to undergo cosmetic surgery to improve your appearance or even your health? If you have, you may be curious about the costs. It is no secret that cosmetic surgery can get costly. However, many individuals, possibly just like you, are more than willing to pay the costs. With that said, do you know how or if you can?

Before getting your heart set on cosmetic surgery, you will want to do a little bit of research first. This research can help you determine how much your cosmetic surgery will cost. With a standard internet search online, you can easily find a few sample rates for common procedures, such as surgical facelifts and liposuction. You can examine these rates, but please know that your local cosmetic surgeons or local cosmetic surgery centers may charge higher rates. Speaking of which, call them. Ask about their rates or see if you should first schedule a consultation appointment

One of the next things that you will want to do is examine your health insurance plan. What coverage are you provided with? Most often, you will find that cosmetic surgery is not covered by a traditional health insurance plan, but you should still look. Why? Because there are some exceptions. For example, some health insurance providers have been known to cover the cost of mole removals and breast reduction surgery.

If your health insurance does not cover the cosmetic surgery procedure you would like to undergo or if you are without health insurance, you will be responsible for the full cost. The best approach to take is to start saving money for your surgery, if you don't already have it. While it may take you awhile, you can set aside a little bit of money each week or each month until you are able to cover the cost of your cosmetic surgery procedure.

In addition to saving money, if you don't already have it, you can inquire about payment plans. Although payment plans do exist, they can be difficult to find. You may also have your credit checked first to make sure that you have a history of making good on your payments. Although it is important for you to be able to afford the cost of cosmetic surgery, especially if you feel like you do not have any other treatment options, it is important to not choose a surgeon or surgical center just based on their availability of a payment plan.

Another option that you have, when looking to pay for your cosmetic surgery, is to pay with a credit card. This is a great approach to take, but be sure to use your best judgment and proceed with caution. Are you good about paying your bill on time? If you are not, the cost of your surgery may significantly increase with late fees. Interest rates may also have an impact on the overcall cost as well.

In all honesty, the best method of payment that you can choose is that of checks or debit cards. This is often the best approach for many. Both checks and debit cards are easy and safe to use and most cosmetic surgeons and cosmetic surgery centers do accept them. As for why checks and debit cards are often the best method of payment, it is because you don't have to carry around large amounts of cash with you. There is a good chance that your surgery will cost a thousand dollars or more.

Now that you know just a few of the many ways that you can go about paying for your cosmetic surgery, you may be ready to move forward. As an important reminder, if you are unable to afford the cost of surgery, examine surgeons and surgical centers that will work to create a payment plan with you, but also make sure that they have a good record with producing quality results and happy patients.

Is Cosmetic Surgery Right for You?

Is cosmetic surgery something that has been on your mind? If might be if you have an imperfection, like excess fat, excess skin, or wrinkles, that you want to fix. As great as cosmetic surgery is, it isn't something that is right for everyone. So, is cosmetic surgery right for you?

The first step in determining if cosmetic surgery is right for you is by examining the cost. Can you afford it? Unless you are going in for reconstructive surgery, like to repair a serious burn or serious cuts and scrapes from an accident, your health insurance provider may not cover the costs. With that said, be sure to check. There are a small number of cosmetic procedures, such as breast reduction surgery, that are occasionally covered and possibly in full. On the back of your health insurance card, there should be a phone number. Call that number and make an inquiry.

Another sign that cosmetic surgery may be right for you is if you are looking to improve your health. Although many individuals opt for cosmetic surgery to only improve their appearance, there are some exceptions. Liposuction and gastric bypass surgery can be used to help you achieve your weight loss goals. Typically, liposuction isn't considered a weight loss plan, like gastric bypass surgery, as you only have around five to ten pounds of fat removed from your problem areas. If you opt for gastric bypass surgery or another similar procedure, you can reduce your risk of heart complications, diabetes, and high blood pressure.

Cosmetic surgery may also be right for you if you don't feel that you have any other options. As it was previously stated, liposuction is ideal for those who have a little bit of extra weight and fat that they would like to have removed. If you have tried eating healthy and exercising, you may not feel like you don't have any options left. The same can be said for slowing the signs of aging. If you have tried numerous over-the-counter products to reduce or eliminate your wrinkles and you haven't seen success, you may see a surgical facelift as your only option. In these instances, cosmetic surgery is usually best.

In keeping with limited options, it is also important to examine that hopelessness you may be feeling. As previously stated, cosmetic surgery is often used to improve one's physical appearance. While you may be told that beauty is more than just your physical appearance, it may have a negative impact on your life. Those who are down or feel like they don't have any other options are likely to suffer from depression, low self-esteem, and have a poor sense of self-confidence. If you are feeling this way, cosmetic surgery is something that is worth looking into.

Perhaps, the most important point to take into consideration is the recovery process. Depending on the cosmetic procedure you undergo, recovery can take a few hours to a few weeks. Be sure to determine this time frame ahead of time. Also, what steps will you need to take to care for yourself? If you undergo a surgical facelift, moisturize or antibiotic cream may need to be applied multiple times a day. Can you remember to do so? If not, cosmetic surgery may not be right for you, as the recovery process can be just as important as the surgery itself.

As a recap, cosmetic surgery is not right for everyone. With that said, if you are looking to improve your self-confidence, your health, and if you can afford the cost of cosmetic surgery, it may be right for you. To see if you are an ideal candidate, contact one of your local cosmetic surgery centers or a surgeon who runs their own private practice. You will want to schedule a consultation appointment. If you are an ideal candidate for surgery, you should get all of the information you need. This information should include a detailed explanation of the procedure, the recovery process, and the total cost.

Laser Hair Removal: The Pros and Cons

Do you have unwanted hair that you would like to have removed? If so, you may be interested in learning more about laser hair removal. Laser hair removal, like all other cosmetic surgery procedures does have its pros and cons.

What many men and women like best about laser hair removal is that the procedure is often considered to be permanent. It honestly depends on how well the job was performed. By taking the time to find a qualified laser surgeon and by following all recovery instructions, you shouldn't have to worry about waxing, shaving, or hiding your unwanted hair anymore.

Another pro or plus side to laser hair removal is that there are little to no side effects. Most individuals will experience a small amount of pain and discomfort, but it is often minimal when compared to other cosmetic procedures. Many also say that laser hair removal is similar to undergoing a waxing procedure. Ask your laser surgeon about the recovery process, like what to do if you experience pain and discomfort. What steps should be taken? Typically, you will find that moisturizing creams, ice packs, and over-the-counter pain medications work best.

The long-term costs are another reason why laser hair removal is a popular choice for men and women, just like yourself. At first glance, the cost of laser hair removal may seem quite high, but it is important to remember that the procedure is long-term. This means that you don't have to spend money on over-the-counter hair removers, shavers and shaving creams, and no more expensive and painful waxing procedures.

Although there are a number of pros or plus sides to undergoing laser hair removal, there are also a number of cons or downsides to doing so as well. One of those is that multiple treatment sessions are needed. As for how many you will have, it will depend on a number of factors. These factors include your gender, skin tone, and the area where work is being performed. Typically, you will find that three to five sessions is the norm.

As highlighted above, cost was sited as a pro to laser hair removal, but it is also important to examine the cost that you are charged. Since you have to undergo multiple treatment sessions, be sure to determine the exact cost. When you call around for information on pricing or when you attend a consultation appoint, get the exact, total cost of treatment. Although laser surgeons rarely offer guarantees, if you are told that only four treatments will be needed, you shouldn't necessarily have to pay for the fifth.

Most importantly, it is important to know that there are risks associated with laser hair removal. These risks may include irritation of the skin, burning of the skin, and scaring. There are, however, ways that you can protect yourself. Don't just choose the laser surgery center that has the cheapest rates. Instead, look for a professional that has affordable rates, yet good qualifications and a high track record of success. Paying a few extra dollars is more than worth it when your risk of complications significantly decreases.

As you can see, there are both a number of pros and cons to laser hair removal. If you are tired of constantly shaving, waxing, or using over-the-counter hair removal products, contact a qualified cosmetic surgeon today. A consultation appointment can help you determine if hair removal by way of laser surgery is your best option.

Popular Cosmetic Dentistry Procedures

Are you looking to improve your appearance? When many of us think of cosmetic improvements, traditional cosmetic surgery procedures, like breast enlargements, facelifts, and liposuction, often come to mind. With that said, those are not the only types of cosmetic surgical procedures you can undergo. If you are looking to improve your smile, namely by way of your teeth, you may want to visit a cosmetic dentist.

As nice as it is to hear that there is such a thing as a cosmetic dentist, who specializes in the appearance of teeth, not just the health of them, you may be looking for more information. One of the most common questions asked concerns procedures. Many wonder what type of cosmetic dentistry procedures are available to them. The good news is that there are quite a few, some of which are briefly highlighted below.

A gum lift is a common cosmetic surgery that is performed by cosmetic dentists. Although most individuals want to change the appearance of their teeth, the teeth aren't always the main problem. If you have uneven or excess gums, your teeth may look uneven and possibly even crooked. If that is the case, a gum lift is advised. During the cosmetic surgical procedure, your excess gum will be removed, giving you an even, flawless smile.

Veneers are another common cosmetic dentistry procedure that is performed. In fact, veneers are increasing in popularity. They are designed for those who have imperfections with their teeth.

These imperfections often include cracked teeth, crooked teeth, or teeth with a significant amount of staining. As for how the procedure works, each tooth will be resized and reshaped. Then, a mold will be taken of the "new," tooth. The dentist's laboratory will then create a custom mold, which will be bonded to your reshaped tooth. Although veneers are a great way to cut down the cost of dental work, please know that they are permanent and that the procedures cannot be reversed.

Another common cosmetic surgical procedure that is performed by qualified dentists is that of dental implants. Do you have a missing tooth or a tooth that needs to be pulled? If you do, dentures may not be a viable option, especially if the rest of your teeth are in healthy shape. If that is the case, dental implants are advised. With dental implants, an artificial tooth is used. That artificial tooth is securely anchored into the jaw bone or the gums. As with veneers, dental implants look and feel just like real teeth.

The above mentioned cosmetic dental procedures are those that can also be considered surgical procedures. It is also important to know that there are additional procedures performed by cosmetic dentists. These procedures are often less invasive and they are typically more affordable. One of those procedures is that of teeth whitening. A professional teeth whitening procedure can reduce stains that are due to coffee, smoking, and aging.

Regardless of how much we all care for our teeth, many of us develop cavities. If you do, the common choice of dentists is that of metal fillings. Ask a cosmetic dentist, however, and they will have a different view. If you are looking to keep your smile and your mouth attractive, you should examine tooth colored fillings. A cosmetic dentist can use a colored coded chart to create the perfect match. Before that is done, however, you may also want to consider undergoing a teeth whitening procedure.

As you can see, you have a number of different options when looking to improve both the health and appearance of your teeth. In fact, the above mentioned procedures are just a few of your many options. You should schedule a consultation appoint with a local, qualified cosmetic dentist to develop an appropriate plan of action. As a reminder, a healthy, beautiful smile can do you wonders. For starters, you will likely notice a significant improvement in your self-esteem and self-confidence.

The Dangers of Cosmetic Surgery

Are you thinking about going under the knife? There is a good chance that you may be. Why? Because cosmetic surgery is increasing in popularity. Many men and women find it to be a relatively easy way to look their best. While this is true in most cases, it is important to know that there are dangers and risks that are associated with cosmetic surgery.

As important as it is to hear that there are dangers and risks associated with cosmetic surgery, that isn't enough to hear. For you to make a well-informed decision, you must also know exactly what those dangers are. Doing so will better allow you to weigh the pros and cons of undergoing cosmetic surgery.

The biggest risk or danger associated with cosmetic surgery is that of pain and discomfort. While not all cosmetic surgery procedures do result in pain and discomfort, a large number of them do. While your pain and discomfort may be able to be treated with over-the-counter pain medicine or an ice pack, it may cut into your daily activities. In fact, the pain may be enough that it could keep you out of work for a couple of days.

Aside from having a small amount of pain and discomfort, there are other side effects to cosmetic surgery. The side effects will depend on the procedure that you have. With that said, another common side effect of cosmetic surgery is that of skin irritation. Your skin will likely be red and it may even feel a little bit itchy. Depending on where on the body your cosmetic surgery was performed, like on your face, you may want to stay indoors or at home for at least a day or two.

Another danger of cosmetic surgery is the chance that complications may arise. This risk is one that many do not necessarily think about because complications are actually quite rare. With that said, it is important to know that they do occur. If you will be given anesthesia and if you know that you are allergic to it or have had reactions to the drug, be sure to tell your surgeon immediately and before the procedure begins.

Another risk that you are taking, when undergoing cosmetic surgery, is that the results may not be what you had hoped for. In fact, every so often you hear reports on the news about how a cosmetic surgeon messed up a patient's procedure, often leaving them worse than they were when they went in for surgery. To reduce the chances of this happening, you will want to be sure that you take the time to find the best cosmetic surgeon or the best cosmetic surgery center in your area. Look for affordable rates, satisfied patients, and a strong surgical background.

In keeping with not getting the results that you had hoped for, it is important to know that you may be stuck with your decision. There are some cosmetic surgery procedures that are difficult, if not impossible to reverse. That is why it is important to make sure that you are sure about your decision to go under the knife. That is also why it is important for you to find a qualified surgeon or surgical center.

It is also important to examine the impact that cosmetic surgery can have on your wallet. There are very few cosmetic procedures that are covered by health insurance. For that reason, you may find yourself responsible for the full cost of your surgery. If that occurs, do you have a plan to come up with the money?

As you can see from being highlighted above, there are a number of dangers and risks that are associated with cosmetic surgery. With that said, it doesn't mean that you should avoid cosmetic surgery at all costs. Instead, it means that you should use your best judgment. Instead of just finding a cheap cosmetic surgeon, find one that has affordable rates, amazing qualifications, and a lot of satisfied patients.

The Importance of Research before Undergoing Cosmetic Surgery

Are you looking to improve your physical appearance? If you are, you may be interested in turning to cosmetic surgery. Many find cosmetic surgery to be a relatively easy and convenient way to remove excess fat from their body, remove excess skin from their body, get a tattoo removed, and slow the signs of aging. Although cosmetic surgery is a great way to improve your appearance, you should first take the time to do the proper amount of research.

As important as it is to hear that you should first research cosmetic surgery before undergoing it, you may be curious as to why you should. In all honestly, there are a number of reasons why you should research cosmetic surgery, namely the specific procedure that you are looking to undergo. For starters, it is easy to do. Second, the decision to undergo cosmetic surgery is a huge decision and it isn't one that should be made on a whim.

Another one of the many reasons why it is important for you to first research cosmetic surgery is because it can help you know what you should expect. While you may already know what you want the end result to be, like a wrinkle-free face, it is important to know how you will get those results. You should never have any surgical procedure done without first knowing exactly what will be done. Reviewing a step-by-step guide is advised.

Researching the cosmetic procedure that you are looking to undergo, like a tummy tuck or a facelift, can also give you an idea of what the recovery process will be like. What you will need to do? Will you need to come back for post recovery checkup or for additional work? Your cosmetic surgeon will provide you with strict recovery instructions, but you may want to research them first. Can you follow the directions? You should be able to, as they may have a significant impact on your health. For example, if you don't properly care for your skin, you may develop a skin infection following your surgery.

Also, researching cosmetic surgery can also give you a good idea as to what the costs will be. Unfortunately, cosmetic surgery can be costly. Is it something that you can afford? Will your health insurance provider cover the cost of your cosmetic surgery? If not, research can help you prepare. For example, if you don't have the needed funds right now, you can get an idea as to how much money you will need to save. Be sure to have some flexibility, as rates do change overtime.

Research can also let you know what the end results of your cosmetic surgery will be. If you are looking to undergo cosmetic surgery to remove your excess skin, after a significant weight loss, you likely know what you want to look like, but will you? Examining before and after pictures are a great way to get a good idea of what you can expect. Of course, you want to look your best, but it is important that you have ideal, realistic expectations.

Now that you know a few reasons why you should first research cosmetic surgery before undergoing it, you may be curious as to how you can do so. For starters, you may want to visit one of your cosmetic surgery centers. They should have pamphlets and other brochures for you to examine. You may also want to set up a consultation appointment. No work will be done, but you can learn about the procedure firsthand

and likely from the doctor who will be performing it.

You can also use the internet to research cosmetic surgery, namely the specific procedure you are looking to undergo. You can get started with a standard internet search. Another approach is to directly visit the online websites of trusted medical companies, like WebMD. When doing so, you know that you are getting accurate and up-to-date information.

The Pros and Cons of Cosmetic Surgery

Have you recently decided that you would like to undergo cosmetic surgery? Whether you are looking to get a tummy tuck, a facelift, or a breast reduction, have you already made your appointment? If this is a step that you have yet to take, you may first want to reexamine your decision. Cosmetic surgery is a big step. Before you move forward, it is important that you examine the pros and cons of going under the knife.

One of the many reasons why cosmetic surgery is so popular is because it has a number of pros or plus sides. For starters, cosmetic surgery can help to improve your appearance. Cosmetic surgery is different than reconstructive surgery and many other lifesaving surgeries, because it is optional. Those who undergo cosmetic surgery are usually just looking to improve their appearance. As nice as it is to look attractive, it is also important to note that you will likely see an improvement in your self-confidence, as well as your self-esteem.

As previously stated, most individuals undergo cosmetic surgery to improve their physical appearance. While this is true, some other individuals do so for their health. Are you overweight or even obese? If you are, cosmetic surgery may actually help to save your life or at least reduce your risk of other health complications, such as high blood pressure and diabetes. Those who are obese are urged to examine the Lapband surgery and gastric bypass surgery. Those who are slightly overweight, but not yet obese, are urged to examine liposuction.

Another pro or plus side to undergoing cosmetic surgery is that it is a convenient option. Yes, you must go into the doctor's office, your procedure may take a few hours, and you may need a few days to recover, but the results are still pretty quick and convenient. For example, if you were looking to remove the excess fat from your arms and thighs, you could spend months or even a year trying to lose the weight through exercise. On the other hand, liposuction will give you the results you wanted, but right away.

Despite the fact that there are a number of pros or plus sides to undergoing cosmetic surgery, it is also important to examine the cons or downsides of it as well. For starters, cosmetic surgery can be costly. The cost will depend on the procedure. A full surgical facelift will cost more money than simply just having a mole removed or the treatment of a stretch mark. Unfortunately, not all health insurance providers cover the cost of cosmetic procedures. In fact, most don't. This means that you will likely be responsible for paying the full cost of your surgery.

Another con or downside to undergoing cosmetic surgery is the risks and dangers that are involved. Side effects, which most often include slight pain and discomfort, are common with most surgical procedures. All surgical procedures, no matter what they are, do have risks. There are no guarantees that you will get the results that you were looking for.

Finally, it is important to examine the recovery process. For many patients, this can be the hardest part. Liposuction was sited as an example above. This surgical procedure is one that has the strictest rules in the recovery process. In addition to letting your body heal, you also need to start eating healthy and exercising. Do you think that you can do so? If not, cosmetic surgery may not be right for you.

As you can see, there are both several pros and cons to undergoing cosmetic surgery. Before you decide to move forward, be sure to thoroughly examine these pros and cons. If you have any additional questions, contact your local cosmetic surgeon or surgical center. In fact, you are urged to first schedule a consultation appointment. Information provided by an experienced cosmetic surgeon can help you reaffirm your decision to go under the knife.

What to Consider When Choosing a Cosmetic Surgery Center

Have you recently decided that you would like to have cosmetic surgery? Whether you are looking to undergo a surgical facelift, a tummy tuck, breast enlargements or reductions, or if you are looking to remove wrinkles and slow the signs of aging, you will need to find a cosmetic surgery center.

As for how you can go about finding a local cosmetic surgery center, you have a number of different options. Those options include performing a standard internet search with your location and the phrase "cosmetic surgery," examining online business directories, using your local phone book, or asking those that you know for recommendations.

Now that you know just a few of the many ways that you can go about finding a local cosmetic surgery center, it is important to know that you need to do more than that. Finding a cosmetic surgery center just isn't good enough; you need to choose one. Why? Because cosmetic surgery can be dangerous and tricky, especially if it is performed by someone with less than stellar qualifications and experience.

So, what should you look for in a quality cosmetic surgery center? For starters, you will want to examine location. Those who wish to undergo cosmetic surgery either go two ways. One, they want to find a local surgery center that is easy and convenient to visit. Second, they want to find the cheapest cosmetic surgery center, even if it means traveling abroad. Depending on where you live, you should be able to find a top-notch cosmetic surgeon within an hour or two of your home.

When looking to choose a cosmetic surgery center, the procedures performed should be examined. What is nice about choosing a cosmetic surgery center, as opposed to one surgeon with a private practice is that you often gain access to the most services and procedures. A cosmetic surgery center is likely to perform a wide range of procedures, even those that involve the use of lasers. With that said, be sure to call ahead and verify first. Also, know that if you are looking to improve your smile, by way of your teeth, a cosmetic dentist should be visited.

Cost is another factor that you should examine, when looking to choose a cosmetic surgery center. Cost is important, as you will not want to be stuck with a surgical procedure that you cannot afford. The first step is examining your health insurance coverage, if you are insured. Is the cosmetic procedure that you would like to undergo covered? If not, you will want to examine alternative methods of payment, which may involve using a credit card, inquiring about payment plans, or taking a few months to save for the surgery.

As important as it is to find a cosmetic surgery center that you can afford, you do not want to lose quality for cost. If you do, you may regret your decision in the end. That is why the reputation of the cosmetic surgery center in question should thoroughly be examined. Do they have a good success rate or a high rate of complications? How much experience do the cosmetic surgeons on staff have? What about training? Would their patients be likely to return again because they were pleased with the results?

Speaking of staffed cosmetic surgeons, will you be able to know ahead of time who is performing your procedure? You should. It isn't a good idea to choose a surgery center that will surprise you on the day of your procedure. Even if a center has a good reputation, please know that the each of the doctors has their own personal amount of work experience, training, and education.

The environment should also be examined. Most reputable cosmetic surgery centers will require you to attend a consultation appointment first. When doing so, how comfortable do you feel in the offices, the waiting room, and in the procedural rooms? Cosmetic surgery is a large step and it is one that some individuals second guess along every step of the way. To prevent this from happening to you, choose a cosmetic surgery center that has a calm, peaceful, relaxing, yet professional environment.

www.ingramcontent.com/pod-product-compliance
Lightning Source LLC
Chambersburg PA
CBHW051213250726
48655CB00006B/2384